Drug and Alcohol Use in Adolescents and Young Adults

ALFRED BROCK

DEDICATION

To all the parents, children and families who are encountering drugs in their communities and schools that they may have a frame of reference to begin with to protect themselves and their loved ones.

CONTENTS

ACKNOWLEDGMENTS

I would like to recognized the CDC (Centers for Disease Control and Prevention), SAMHSA (the Substance Abuse and Mental Health Service Administration and NIDA (National Institute or. Drug Abuse)

All three of these fine organizations have compiled information about the dangers of drug use and abuse and make it freely available.

I recommend that you visit them at your first opportunity and use this book as a reference as you seek answers to your questions about drug use and what to do about it.

INTRODUCTION

In the United States today there is a drug overdose epidemic. It is wounding and killing many people, especially young people. They can freely access a wide variety of powerful drugs. These drugs can have profound life changing consequences.

Use of these drugs can lead to addiction where the person using them needs to replenish their supply regularly or they will become sick. This resupply activity can become extremely expensive. If the money is not available for someone to purchase the drugs they may turn to criminal activities to get them. Some people exploit (sell) themselves to get a supply of the drugs they are seeking.

These drugs can also be adulterated, or have things added to them, that make them even more dangerous. The addition of fentanyl, for example, to drugs like heroin and cocaine, can lead to lifelong disability or death.

Many of the people purchasing and using these drugs, especially adolescents, are unaware of the potency of these drugs.

All of the substances in this book are poisonous if enough of them are taken. They can become poisonous at lower doses if mixed with other drugs and substances.

This is a complex issue with no quick fix once the problem has started. There are ways, however, to detect drug use early enough to intercede in a positive fashion with what is going on and even stop it before it goes too far. This is a job for individuals, families and friends. It is a community issue and we will all need to work together to solve it. The important thing is that you are not alone.

Older adults and seniors are not immune to this problem. As the illegal drug problem has worsened the availability of more and more powerful drugs used in medicine has increased as well. Older Americans are now prescribed powerful narcotics. These drugs can and do cause problems in their lives. By being aware of potential problems and symptoms we can help ourselves and our seniors enjoy life without being overcome by drugs first intended to help them.

This book can be used by all ages. It is intended as a guide to allow people to detect drug use in other – especially their loved ones. Drug use can go undetected until it has become a serious problem. After a drug problem has been revealed and steps taken to mitigate it or stop it then detecting ongoing drug use becomes even more critical.

Drug use can be easily hidden. This is not an exhaustive set of directions for detecting drug use. If a person wants to hide their drug use they can find ways to do it. The marketplace helps them along as we shall see. There are many products for sale today specifically targeting drug uses, and young drug users at that, to help them hide their drugs and conceal their drug use.

This book is arranged in four parts.

The first part deals with the various drugs that are abused in the United States. Details on the drug are provided along with their names and common names. Information about Detecting use of that particular drug are provided as well.

HOW TO USE THIS BOOK

In the first portion of the book each drug will be presented.

There will be technical information about the drug along with ways that the drug is used.

The effects of the drug will also be listed.

Through all of the descriptions of the drugs and their impacts the words that are used to describe them by dealers and user will occur in the text.

The terminology is provided to allow those screening for the use of these drugs in loved ones, their friends or acquaintances as audio cues to pick up on what is being discussed.

Often, when drug users do not have their guard up they will freely use drug related jargon to communicate about drugs, their uses, availability and other things.

This is a very important aspect of detecting drug use but one that changes rapidly.

Individual drugs have their street names changed on a regular basis and from time to time specific lots of drugs are given a name by dealers or drug users.

CHAPTER 1

METHAMPHETAMINE USE

What is methamphetamine?

"Methamphetamine is a powerful, highly addictive stimulant that affects the central nervous system. Crystal methamphetamine is a form of the drug that looks like glass fragments or shiny, bluish-white rocks. It is chemically similar to amphetamine, a drug used to treat attention-deficit hyperactivity disorder (ADHD) and narcolepsy, a sleep disorder.

Other common names for methamphetamine include blue, crystal, ice, meth, and speed."

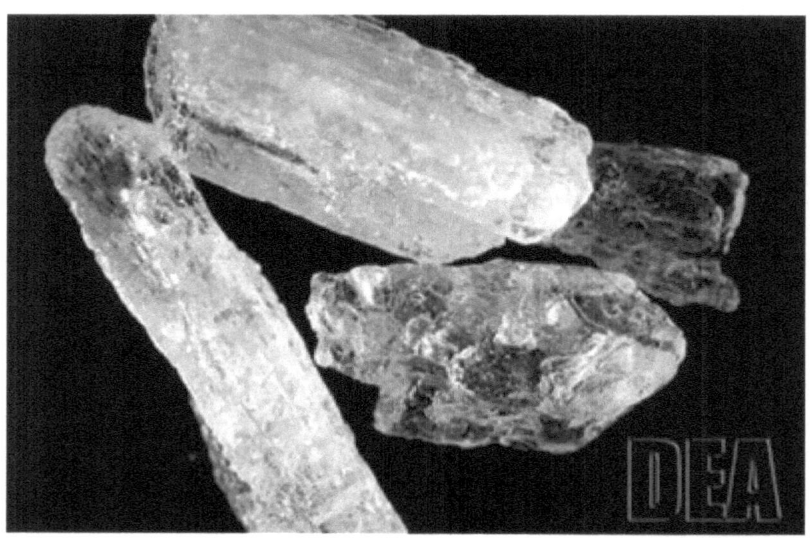

Courtesy of DrugFacts

People use methamphetamine by:

smoking
swallowing (pill)
snorting (through the nose)

injecting the powder that has been dissolved in water/alcohol Because the "high" from the methamphetamine is relatively brief, people often use it in a "binge and crash" way. Sometimes methamphetamine is taken in a pattern known as a "run". The user will even give up food and sleep to use the drug every few hours.

This can go on for days.

Methamphetamines are a highly addictive stimulant that can be smoked, injected, inhaled or taken by mouth. Symptoms of meth abuse include:

increased attention and decreased fatigue
increased activity and wakefulness
increased talkativeness
decreased appetite
euphoria
increased respiration
rapid/irregular heartbeat
hyperthermia

Methamphetamine's main effect is that it artificially increases the amount of the natural chemical dopamine in the brain. This Dopamine is necessary for body movement, motivation, and the reinforcement of rewarding behaviors. Even though there is no physical or mental reward provided by the drug the sensation of that false reward is what drives its use. The drug forces the rapid release of incredibly high levels of dopamine in reward areas of the brain. The person being then inebriated identifies only with the sensation and repeatedly administers it until the supply runs out, they pass out, become incapacitated or die.

Several signs that a person may be using methamphetamines. The physical appearance and behavior of a person using methamphetamines is a good place to start.

Skin picking: methamphetamine addicts are known to obsessively pick at their skin. The marks left by this picking may look similar to an extreme case of acne, often leaving open sores on the face.

Skin crawling: meth addicts also often complain about having crawling skin, a disorder known as formication.

Tooth decay: Another common sign is tooth loss or tooth decay that drug users have come to refer to as meth mouth.

Hair loss: due to the lack of nutrients in an addict's body as well as the dangerous chemicals they ingest, hair breakage and loss frequently occurs as well.

In addition, methamphetamine users can develop other symptoms. They are very similar to Parkinson's disease, which is a severe movement disorder.

As the body requires calcium to detoxify amphetamines, many users develop trouble with teeth, gums, fingernails, and dry lifeless hair.

Those who inject methamphetamine increase their risk of contracting infectious diseases such as HIV, Hepatitis B and C and others.

The diseases are transmitted through contact with blood or other bodily fluids that can remain on drug equipment.

The social structure around the use of Methamphetamine and the drug itself alters judgment and decision-making which leads to risky behavior. Unprotected sex, one of these behaviors also increases risk for infection and disease.

Methods of Methamphetamine use include many forms. The substance can be smoked, snorted, injected or eaten.

Methamphetamine use methods vary over time due to the type of material being made or imported into the area, availability of devices like specialty pipes, syringes, powders or pills.

The smoking of methamphetamine, often mixed with other substances like cigarettes, marijuana or other drugs is common. If a child is smoking cigarettes or has other smoking paraphernalia in their possession it is not unreasonable to be wary of methamphetamines being a danger. Methamphetamines become addictive quickly. They are especially worrisome as they come along with a heavy psychological addiction. The physical addiction can be over with fairly quickly, however, the psychological addiction can persist for some time. This is also due in no small way to the bizarre social settings in which it is used, encouraged, bought and sold.

Tolerance increases quickly. There will be a swift change in behavior and getting money to pay for the substance may rapidly become an issue.

Methamphetamines cause :
       Impaired judgment
       Suspiciousness
       Aggressive behavior
       Violent behavior
       Loss of sleep
       Suppression of appetite

Long term impacts from the use of methamphetamines include :
       Memory loss
       Psychotic behavior
       Moderate to severe espiratory problems
       Loss of weight
       Brain damage
       Stroke
       Heart damage
       Death
       Acne

Withdrawal from methamphetamines, caused either by a lack of the drug or intentionally stopping use, can cause :
       Depression
       Suicidal ideation and attempts
       Excessive fatigue
       Fluctuating appetite

A strong desire to possess and use the drug
Methamphetamine withdrawal symptoms, like most drug
withdrawal symptoms, are not life threatening. Severe depression,
suicidal ideation and attempts can be. If this is a possibility or
becomes one during withdrawal then hospitalization and
professional care should be provided immediately.

Consult with your physician for further information.
Where do methamphetamines come from?

It is reported at this time that a majority methamphetamine in the
United States is produced by transactional criminal organizations
(TCOs) in Mexico.

This methamphetamine is highly pure, potent, and low in price.
The drug is easily made in small laboratories. The ingredients and
equipment to make it with is inexpensive. Over-the-counter
ingredients include pseudoephedrine which is a common
ingredient in cold medications.

To slow this kind of manufacturing pharmacies and other stores
have to keep a purchase record of products containing
pseudoephedrine and limit sales.

Methamphetamine production involves other dangerous chemicals.
Toxic effects from these chemicals can and do persist in the
environment long after the laboratory stops production. These
chemicals cause many health problems for others living in the area.
The chemicals can also cause lab explosions and house fires that
can kill the producers, dealers, users and bystanders.

An important note to make is that if someone breathes in
secondhand smoke from methamphetamines they can test positive
for having used the drug.

In the year 2017 around 15 percent of drug overdose deaths in the
United States involved methamphetamines. Of those 50 percent
included an opioid and then half of those deaths were related to
fentanyl.

Cheap, dangerous opioids and other drugs and chemicals are sometimes added to methamphetamines without the knowledge of the person using it.

Most methamphetamine overdoses lead to a stroke, heart attack, or organ problems. First responders and emergency room doctors try to treat the overdose by treating these conditions. They try to restore blood flow to the affected part of the brain for a stroke. For a heart attack they attempt to restore blood flow to the heart. There are other things they attempt for other organ problems that can occur.

Anywhere in the process of using methamphetamine a person may lose consciousness, lack oxygen and experience mini-strokes, minor heart attacks and organ damage that they may be unaware of. Over time their ability to think, understand, learn, and remember will be damaged. The overall destruction of the body and mind leads to or brings to the surface mental and emotional problems.

Studies suggest methamphetamine may cause structural and functional changes in the brain. These changes are those that have been associated with emotion and memory.

Some of these may be irreversible.

Portions of this material were adapted from :
Source: National Institute on Drug Abuse; National Institutes of Health; U.S. Department of Health and Human Services.

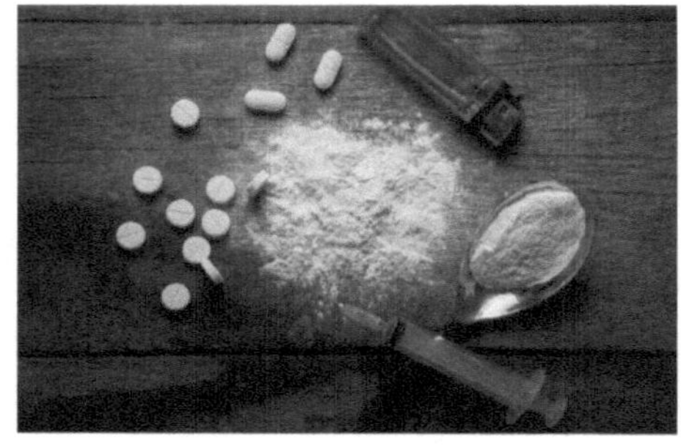

Drug	Time Period	8th Graders	10th Graders	12th Graders
Methamphetamine	Lifetime	0.90	0.70	0.80
	Past Year	0.50	0.50	0.50
	Past Month	0.10	0.30	0.30

Monitoring the Future Study: Trends in Prevalence of Methamphetamine for 8th Graders, 10th Graders, and 12th Graders; 2019 (in percent)*

Drug	Time Period	Ages 12 or Older	Ages 12 to 17	Ages 18 to 25	Ages 26 or Older
Methamphetamine	Lifetime	5.40	0.30	2.50	6.50
	Past Year	0.70	0.20	0.80	0.70
	Past Month	0.40	0.10	0.30	0.40

National Survey on Drug Use and Health: Trends in Prevalence of Methamphetamine for Ages 12 or Older, Ages 12 to 17, Ages 18 to 25, and Ages 26 or Older; 2018 (in percent)*

Table 1. Ingredients Used in the Production of Meth.

Alcohol	Hydrochloric/muriatic acid
Anhydrous ammonia-fertilizer	Hydrogen peroxide
Antifreeze	Iodine crystals
Battery acid	Lead acetate
Benzene	Lighter fluid
Charcoal lighter fluid	Lithium from batteries
Diet aids/ephedrine	Lye-sodium hydroxide
Di-ethyl ether – camp stove fuel	Nail polish remover – acetone
Energy boosters	OTC cold medicine/pseudoephedrine

Ethyl ether – starter fluid	Paint thinner
Freon	Red phosphorus – matches/flares
Gasoline	Sulfuric acid – drain cleaner

Table 2. Equipment Used in the Production of Meth.

Gas cans	Pails/buckets
Hot plates	Propane cylinders
Ice chests	Rubber gloves
Jugs and bottles	Rubber tubing
Kitty litter	Tempered glassware
Laboratory beakers/glassware	Thermometers

Current common names for methamphetamines include :
Speed, Crank, Chalk, Wash, Trash, Dunk, Gak, Pookie, Cookies, Christina, No doze, White cross, Cotton candy, Rocket fuel, Scooby snax

There are also several slang terms for the act of getting high by taking meth. These can include:
Getting geared up, Chicken flipping, Hot rolling, Getting fried or foiled, Tweaking, Zooming, Getting scattered or spun out

Meth can also be mixed with other illicit drugs in order to intensify its effects or to alter the effects of other intoxicants. Common slang names for these combinations include:
Fire, Shabu, Twisters, Hugs and kisses, Biker coffee, Party and play

CHAPTER 2

OPIOID USE

In the present day United States opioids are dispensed at an alarming rate. You, or someone you know, may have some in your home right now. This set of drugs is very powerful and very dangerous.

Prescription opioids are derived either directly from organic opioids or contain some portion of them. Many of them are equivalent to heroin. Several of them, including fentanyl and carfentenil are much more powerful. All of them have the properties necessary to induce dependence in the human body and ultimately addiction.

Opioids have become a danger in the United States. Up until the 1980's they were used only in the most severe cases of pain such as in end-of-life treatment and on the battle field.

In the United States today opioids are used to mask pain following surgery or injury and for cancer. Prescriptions have been made in the present day for a many more reasons. The definition of an injury that can be treated with opioids expanded from broken and torn limbs to sprains and bruises. Opioids have been provided to teenagers and adults in amounts that spur dependence and in some case enough to cause addiction.

Often the opioids are dispensed without the information necessary to know that they can have profound life-changing effects and may cause addiction and death.

From the CDC :

"More than 191 million opioid prescriptions were dispensed to American patients in 2017—with wide variation across states.1

There is a wide variation of opioid prescription rates across states. Health care providers in the highest prescribing state, Alabama, wrote almost three times as many of these prescriptions per person as those in the lowest prescribing state, Hawaii.1

Studies suggest that regional variation in use of prescription opioids cannot be explained by the underlying health status of the population.2

The most common drugs involved in prescription opioid overdose deaths include:

Methadone

Oxycodone (such as OxyContin®)

Hydrocodone (such as Vicodin®)"

As we know any human being who takes prescription opioids can become addicted. About 25% of all patients provide long-term opioid prescriptions in a primary care setting end up struggling with opioid addiction. Out patient treatment that includes 30 to 60 to 90 pills will also cause dependence and ultimately addiction if all the pills are consumed. Depending on how long the opioid use is and at what level withdrawal symptoms will occur even with a small amount of the drug. Withdrawal symptoms are normally over within 5 to 7 days.

There is a lot of folklore and horror stories that go along with withdrawal symptoms that is shared among drug users and encouraged by the dealers. The specter of withdrawal is much more frightening than the reality which can last 5 to 7 days and be equal to a very bad cold or the flu. Depending on the person's body type, physical condition and amount of use they may experience a great deal of pain and anxiety. Many people choose to stop using opioids on their own and successfully get through the withdrawal portion but fail again after time due to habit, keeping the same social circle and visiting places where the drugs are available.

Once being physically addicted it can be hard to stop. In 2016, more than eleven and a half mllion Americans reported misusing prescription opioids that year. This is truly an epidemic.

Many drug users believe that just because it is a prescription opioid made by a pharmaceutical company that the pills are safe. This is not true. Taking too many prescription opioids can kill. It does this in the same way that illegal forms of opioids. They slow the heart rate and respiration to such a point that they stop and the person dies.

We will learn more about benzodiazepines later but please be aware that many opioid overdose deaths also include benzodiazepines. Benzodiazepines are central nervous system depressants that are supposed to be used to sedate, induce sleep, prevent seizures, and relieve anxiety. Examples of these pills are alprazolam (Xanax®), diazepam (Valium®), and lorazepam (Ativan®).

Anyone using opioids should not be taking benzodiazepines. It is a dangerous combination and can result in mental and physical disability or death.

Even when taken as directed along with the dangerous risk of addiction, abuse, and overdose, the use of prescription opioids can have a number of side effects :

Tolerance—meaning you might need to take more of the medication for the same pain relief

Physical dependence—meaning you have symptoms of withdrawal when the medication is stopped or even slowed

There will be an increased sensitivity to pain

Constipation will occur with all sorts of opioids and is a major complaint of users

Nausea, vomiting, and dry mouth

Sleepiness and dizziness

Confusion

Depression

Low levels of testosterone that can result in lower sex drive, energy, and strength

Itching and sweating

Drug	Time Period	8th Graders	10th Graders	12th Graders
Heroin	Past Year	0.30	0.30	0.40
Narcotics other than Heroin	Past Year	-	-	[2.70]
OxyContin	Past Year	1.20	2.00	1.70
Vicodin	Past Year	0.90	1.10	[1.10]

Monitoring the Future Study: Trends in Prevalence of Various Drugs for 8th Graders, 10th Graders, and 12th Graders; 2019 (in percent)*

Drug	Time Period	Ages 12 or Older	Ages 12 to 17	Ages 18 to 25	Ages 26 or Older
Heroin	Past Year	0.30	0.00	0.50	0.30
Pain Relievers	Past Year	3.60	2.80	5.50	3.40

National Survey on Drug Use and Health: Trends in Prevalence of Various Drugs for Ages 12 or Older, Ages 12 to 17, Ages 18 to 25, and Ages 26 or Older; 2018 (in percent)*

Any time it has been determined that a person has had an opioid overdose it is important to call 9-1-1 first.

If caught in time an opioid overdose can be reversed with the drug naloxone. Depending on the circumstances it may take more than one dose of naloxone to revive someone from an opioid overdose. Even if this is done in time it is critical for the person to receive medical attention. The reason for this is that naloxone does not last as long as opioids in the blood and body. If the naloxone is used up then the overdose will continue and disability or death may occur.

The misuse of opioids by teenagers and young adults is troubling. They are often given access to these powerful drugs without knowing the consequences. Whether they began receiving them for an injury or some medical procedure or from friends or family makes no difference. The impact is the same. It can lead to dependence, addiction and disability and death in a short time or turn a fine life into a terrible ordeal.

There are some other drugs used to treat opioid addiction, if the person cannot escape the drug alone. These include methadone, buprenorphine and naltrexone.

 Improvements have been seen in some regions of the country in the form of decreasing availability of prescription opioid pain relievers and decreasing misuse among the Nation's teens. However, since 2007, overdose deaths related to heroin have been increasing. Fortunately, effective medications exist to treat opioid use disorders including methadone, buprenorphine, and naltrexone.

These three drugs are not magic. They come with their own set of cautions and warnings. It is best to avoid opioids rather than having later to withdraw from them and possibly need these other drugs to stay alive.

Naltrexone warnings include :

May cause dizziness

This drug may impair the ability to operate a vehicle, vessel (e.g., boat), or machinery. Use care until you become familiar with its effects.

If you are pregnant or considering becoming pregnant you should discuss the use of this medication with your doctor or pharmacist.

Call your doctor immediately if you have mental/mood changes like confusion, new/worsening feelings of sadness/fear, thoughts of suicide, or unusual behavior.

Opioids should be avoided at all costs when using Naltrexone as they cause the person taking it to not feel the effects of opioids. Though they cannot feel the effects of any opioids they may take the opioids will still act upon the body and brain causing disability or death.

Methadone warnings include :

CAUTION: Opioid. Risk of overdose and addiction.

May cause drowsiness and dizziness. Alcohol and marijuana may intensify this effect. Use care when operating a vehicle, vessel (e.g., boat), or machinery.

If you are pregnant or of childbearing age, discuss the risks/benefits of this medication with your doctor and pharmacist.

Do not drink alcoholic beverages when using this medication.

Using more of this medication than recommended may cause serious breathing problems.

Do not share this drug with others. This amount of drug may cause serious toxicity or harm if used by someone not used to this much drug.

Buprenorphine warnings include :

If pregnant or of childbearing age the risks/benefits of this medication should be discussed at length with your doctor and pharmacist.

May cause drowsiness and dizziness. Alcohol and marijuana may intensify this effect. Use care when operating a vehicle, vessel (e.g., boat), or machinery.

Do not drink alcoholic beverages when using this medication.

Using more of this medication than recommended may cause serious breathing problems.

Keep in refrigerator. Do not freeze.

Bring to room temperature before preparing for use.

CAUTION: Ask your doctor before using this drug with other opioids, sleep or anxiety drugs, or other drugs that can cause serious breathing problems/drowsiness.

"A NIDA study found that once treatment is initiated, both a buprenorphine/naloxone combination and an extended release naltrexone formulation are similarly effective in treating opioid addiction. However, naltrexone requires full detoxification, so initiating treatment among active users was more difficult. These medications help many people recover from opioid addiction."

From the National Institute on Drug Abuse (NIDA)

Heroin is an opioid drug derived in a laboratory from morphine. Morphine is derived from opium which is a natural substance taken from the seed pod of the various opium poppy plants grown in Southeast and Southwest Asia, Mexico, and Colombia.

Heroin can be a white or brown powder, or a black sticky substance known as black tar heroin. Common names for heroin include big H, horse, hell dust, and smack.

The uses of heroin include injecting, sniffing, snorting or smoking it. Sometimes people mix heroin with crack cocaine in a practice called speedballing. The drug is often adulterated with other materials as it makes its way down the marketing change from producer to user.

The Short-Term Effects of Heroin include :

People who use heroin report feeling a "rush" (a surge of pleasure, or euphoria). However, there are other common effects, including:

dry mouth

warm flushing of the skin

heavy feeling in the arms and legs

nausea and vomiting

severe itching

clouded mental functioning

going "on the nod," a back-and-forth state of being conscious and semiconscious

Cocaine, methamphetamines and other stimulants can cause a stroke to occur in two ways. The first is that stimulant drugs increase blood pressure. These drugs have an immediate and direct effect on blood vessel walls. Increased pressure can cause them to burst and blood leaks into the brain. This stroke type is referred to as a hemorrhagic.

The same stimulant drugs cause blood vessels to become narrower. This can lead to the prevention of normal blood flow to parts of the brain and therefore destroys brain tissue. This stroke type is referred to as an ischemic stroke.

The Long-Term Effects of Heroin include :

insomnia

collapsed veins for people who inject the drug

damaged tissue inside the nose for people who sniff or snort it

infection of the heart lining and valves

abscesses (swollen tissue filled with pus)

constipation and stomach cramping

liver and kidney disease

lung complications, including pneumonia

mental disorders such as depression and antisocial personality disorder

sexual dysfunction for men

irregular menstrual cycles for women

constipation

Other potential impacts from the user of heroin include :

Heroin often contains additives, such as sugar, starch, or powdered milk, that can clog blood vessels leading to the lungs, liver, kidneys, or brain, causing permanent damage.

Sharing drug injection equipment and having impaired judgment from drug use can increase the risk of contracting infectious diseases such as HIV, hepatitis and other diseases.

When people overdose on heroin breathing slows or stops. This decreases the oxygen that reaches the brain which is a condition known as hypoxia.

Hypoxia can have both short- and long-term mental effects and impact the nervous system, including the onset of a coma and permanent brain damage.

Heroin is highly addictive and causes a tolerance. This means they need more of the drug to get the imagined effects.

A substance use disorder (SUD) happens when the drug causes health problems and failure to meet responsibilities at work, school, or home.

Withdrawal symptoms—which can begin as early as a few hours after the drug was last taken—include:

restlessness

severe muscle and bone pain

sleep problems

diarrhea and vomiting

cold flashes with goose bumps ("cold turkey")

uncontrollable leg movements ("kicking the habit")

severe heroin cravings

anxiety

tearing and dilated pupils

runny nose

excessive sweating

insomnia

yawning

goose bumps

rapid heartbeat and high blood pressure

These symptoms can be very uncomfortable and through word of mouth and assurances by dealers the general idea has been planted in drug society that withdrawal is dangerous.

How to tell if someone is abusing opioids :

It may not be that easy to tell. In the early stages of addiction everything can look and seem normal.

As time goes on behavior and circumstances may change. These may take place slowly over time so a watchful eye and a kind heart can go a long way. If the person wishes to they may begin to hide their addiction and lie about it. Tips on what is going on would be missing money, possessions, disorientation, stories that don't make sense, restlessness, anger and aggressive behavior. Even these more serious developments may seem normal if the change takes place over time.

Some points to keep in mind about the danger of addiction to anyone are :

The person in their teens or early 20s

The person is living in stressful circumstances, including being unemployed or living below the poverty line

The person already has a personal or family history of substance abuse

Is exhibiting now or has had a history of problems with work, family and friends

Has experienced legal problems including DUIs

In in the habit of hanging out with or is in regular contact with high-risk people or high-risk environments where there's drug use

The person has struggled with or is struggling with severe depression or anxiety

The person may tend to engage in risk-taking or thrill-seeking behavior

The person is a heavy user of tobacco

Signs of opioid use and addiction include:

Regularly taking an opioid in a way not intended by the doctor who prescribed it, including taking more than the prescribed dose or taking the drug for the way it makes a person feel

Taking opioids "just in case," even when not in pain

Mood changes that include excessive swings from elation to hostility

Changes in sleep patterns

Borrowing medication from other people or "losing" medications so that more prescriptions must be written

Seeking the same prescription from multiple doctors, in order to have a "backup" supply

Poor decision-making, including putting himself or herself and others in danger

A person addicted to opioids or any drugs including alcohol is much more likely to recover if his or her family refuses to ignore or tolerate the problem.

CHAPTER 3

COCAINE USE

Cocaine is a highly addictive drug that increases metabolism, narrows attention and creates frenetic physical and mental activity. Sometimes it is called a stimulant.

It has restricted medical uses but generally has fallen out of favor for other drugs that provide the same work without the unnecessary side effects.

The drug is extracted from the coca plant. The coca plant is native to high elevations. The plant's leaves and other parts have been used by Native American in South America for centuries. The plant's leaves have a mild narcotic and stimulant effect, that, nonetheless, even though it is mild, becomes addictive over time.

After the coca leaves are picked they are mulched in large piles.

After this they are treated with cement to help them stick together and make coca paste. The coca paste preparation continues in large vats where gasoline, ether and other chemicals are mixed in. Other chemicals include ammonia, sulfuric acid, sodium permanganate and caustic soda. The next step involves using hydrochloric acide, alcohol, ammonia, acetone, laboratory equipment and a microwave.

A coca farmer earns about $1000 a year on average.

The chemist who makes the cocaine from the paste makes about $830 per kilo.

At the first stop in Columbia the cost for a kilo of cocaine is about $1456.

At the border it increases to $4000 per kilo.

In the United States a kilo can cost about $33600.

In Germany the price surges to over $400,000 a kilo.

Other names for cocaine include:

> Coke
> Snow
> Rock
> Blow
> Crack

It can be turned into different kinds of cocaine. The common one is a white powder. Later processing can turn into larger crystals.

Cocaine is usually inhaled through the nose in a process known as 'snorting.' Some people rub it in their gums and mouth, dissolve it in water and inject it with a needle. Application to genitals is very dangerous and can lead to heart attack and death especially with women. Sometimes the crystallized form of the drug is heated and the resulting smoke is breathed in.

How It Works

The drug spurs the brain to release unnatural amounts of dopamine. Dopamine functions both as a hormone and a neurotransmitter and performs several important functions in the brain and the rest of the body.

At this point the drug is actually poisoning the body by forcing it to do something unnatural. The length of time it takes for the drug to cause deleterious effects like destroying organs and the mind is dependent on the person and the amount and type of the drug that is ingested. No one is immune to the poisonous effects of cocaine.

After the first time or the first few times of the use of cocaine the effect of confused gaiety and muscle activity quickly descends in mere hunger for the drug. Each subsequent use required more of the drug to achieve imagined effects. The effects do not last but the impact of the drug on the body does persist.

The short-term effects of cocaine use include constriction of the blood vessels, dilated pupils, increased body temperature, heart rate and higher blood pressure.

Large amounts of cocaine can cause bizarre, erratic, and violent behavior.

Cocaine often creates feelings of restlessness, irritability, anxiety, panic, and paranoia along with tremors, vertigo, and muscle twitches.

Long-term use can alter the mind and body and damage both of them. The cardiovascular is often negatively impacted leading to disturbances in heart rhythm and heart attacks. Neurological impacts can also happen and include headaches, seizures, strokes, and coma.

Gastrointestinal complications which can include abdominal pain and nausea often also develop. This causes a person using cocaine to stop or reduce eating. Some users claim it is a great drug to use in order to lose weight but the reason weight loss occurs is because the gastrointestinal system is poisoned and damaged and eating and digesting food becomes painful.

On occasions sudden death can occur on the first use of cocaine or within a short time afterward.

Cocaine deaths are often a result of cardiac arrest or seizures.

Cocaine users also consume alcohol when taking the drug. The mixing of these two drugs is dangerous. Together cocaine and alcohol create cocaethylene in the body. This toxin has increases the toxicity of cocaine and alcohol on the heart.

Come cocaine users also combine cocaine with heroin in another very dangerous mix. They do this as the common parlance has it that it the stimulating effects of cocaine are offset by the sedating effects of heroin. What happens is that when cocaine is imbibed the body demands more oxygen. When heroin is taken the body's respiration is decrease. Just as the cocaine is overstimulating the body to demand more oxygen the heroin is decreasing the oxygen level. Heart attack or a situation akin to drowning in air can occur and breathing stops. If a person is not revived within three to nine minutes and provided medical treatment irreversible brain damage can occur. If the time to resuscitation is longer than that that death may occur and is most likely.

Other difficulties that cocaine users can experience include :

> Headaches
> Convulsions and seizures
> Heart disease, heart attack, and stroke
> Mood problems
> Sexual trouble
> Lung damage
> HIV or hepatitis through sharing of drug equipment, close proximity and sex
> Gangrenous bowl and perforation of the bowels
> Loss of smell, nosebleeds, runny nose, and trouble swallowing, if you snort it

Cocaine, methamphetamines and other stimulants can cause a stroke to occur in two ways. The first is that stimulant drugs increase blood pressure. These drugs have an immediate and direct effect on blood vessel walls. Increased pressure can cause them to burst and blood leaks into the brain. This stroke type is referred to as a hemorrhagic.

The same stimulant drugs cause blood vessels to become narrower. This can lead to the prevention of normal blood flow to parts of the brain and therefore destroys brain tissue. This stroke type is referred to as an ischemic stroke.

Following even brief use of cocaine people who take it may experience strong cravings for the drug. These cravings can, and often do, begin to interfere with normal human relations including those with family and friends. In order to get the drug people who take it often change their social circumstances and people associated with the drug rather than with other interests begin to become dominant in their lives.

The more cocaine is used the more changes that will occur in the brain and body. Dependence and addiction sets in rather quickly after which the circumstances for an overdose are at hand at each and every use.

Cocaine changes a person's physical and mental makeup. It will become harder for them to think, sleep, and recall things from memory. Comprehension will drop.
Reaction time, though perceived by the user to quicken, will slow.

The user is at risk for more heart, stomach, and lung problems and will begin to exhibit symptoms early on that indicate that a once healthy individual is suffering from long-term ailments usually encountered by older people and senior.

Counseling and other various different types of therapy are treatments for cocaine addiction. The person may need to stay in a rehabilitation center or decide to go there. Depending on which one is chosen the cost can be very high. Families that have attempted to help and who have helped family members through this time may experience financial hardship or bankruptcy.

Changes in behavior and thought processes are necessary. Medical and psychological problems that existed can be made worse by the drug or medical and psychological problems may be caused by the drug. The society from which the drugs come from and where the person using cocaine spends time also causes problems of their own. The ideas and directions provided to someone using cocaine by those selling cocaine are often abusive and deceptive.

CHAPTER 4

BENZODIAZEPINE USE

Benzodiazepines are psychoactive drugs used to treat different things which include anxiety and insomnia.

These drugs are some of the most widely prescribed medications in the United States. They are especially prescribed often to older patients. Their use in the drug culture, however, has assured that a large supply moves into the hands of underage and illegal users and distributors.

Benzodiazepines can help to reduce anxiety and seizures, relax muscles, and make people to to sleep.

Short-term use of these medications is considered generally safe and effective though for some people it can prove to be a problem. As for long-term use they become increasingly dangerous because tolerance rises and dependence can appear. Other bad health impacts come along with their use.

They are very powerful drugs and taking enough of them can cause an overdose as what were supposed to be helpful benefits go to far and produce poisonous results. Mixing benzodiazepines with alcohol, cocaine, opioids and other things can lead to lifelong disability or death.

Benzodiazepines affect the brain by stimulating an unnatural level of a chemical in the brain that causes a tranquilizing condition.

Side effects of this drug can include :

Dizziness

Lack of coordination

Depression

Trembling

Amongst older users it appears that there is an increased risk of dementia

Hospital admissions for benzodiazepine use have increased dramatically in the past twenty years.

The drugs have been approved to be used to treat insomnia, generalized anxiety disorders, some seizures, alcohol withdrawal: The most common benzodiazepine prescribed for alcohol withdrawal is chlodiazepoxide, followed by diazepam. The drugs help people with alcohol dependence by removing toxins from their system and reducing the risk of severe alcohol withdrawal symptoms and panic attacks. Though it has been approved for these uses there are groups of doctors that do not believe that benzodiazepines should be used for panic attacks.

There are many commercial types of benzodiazepines and these include, but are not limited to :

Alprazolam or Xanax, Chlordiazepoxide or Librium, Clorazepate or Tranxene, Diazepam or Valium, Estazolam, Flurazepam or Dalmane, Oxazepam, Temazepam or Restoril, Triazolam or Apo-Triazo, Halcion, Hypam, and Trilam.

The drugs seem mild but withdrawal symptoms from occur and include trouble sleeping, feelings of depression, and sweating. They can also become life threatening as stopping without tapering off these powerful drugs can bring on severe tremors, painful muscle cramps and life-threatening seizures.

Overdose is severe danger with benzodiazepines especially if mixed with alcohol, cocaine or opioids.

Some other drugs like antidepressant and oral contraceptives can cause a dangerous buildup of medications within the body. These effects can worsen the side effects of benzodiazepines.

Along with the fact that these drugs can abused by drug users they can also be used as a poison in order to take advantage of people including robbery and rape.

Benzodiazepines are used as a "date rape" drug. They can impair and even remove actions in the body and mind that normally allow a person to resist or even want to resist sexual aggression or assault.

In the past twenty years the number of people involved in these heinous crimes has increased greatly. The drug is added to alcohol drinks or soft drinks in powder or liquid forms. When the poison is given in this way it can be hard to taste.

Withdrawal from benzodiazepines can cause severe anxiety and panic attacks, insomnia, depression, irritability, aggression, confusion, depersonalization in a sense that the person feels they are not real or has no identity. There is also a strong danger of ideation and actions towards suicide.

These drugs are often bought, sold and used in pill, power or liquid form. They are generally easy to conceal and the user may be able to hide their use for some time.

Comparisons between past behaviors and present behaviors with knowledge about what would be expected behavior from a similar person at a similar age and in similar circumstances may help in identifying use but is not guaranteed.

CHAPTER 5

MARIJUANA USE

Marijuana is the dried leaves, flowers, stems, and seeds from the Cannabis sativa or Cannabis indica plants. The plants contain the mind-altering chemical THC (tetrahydrocannabinol) and other similar chemical compounds. Extracts are also commonly made from the cannabis plant.

People smoke the THC-rich resins extracted from the marijuana plant. Some people call this "dabbing". The extracts can be :
hash oil or honey oil—a gooey liquid
wax or budder—a soft solid with a texture like lip balm
shatter—a hard, amber-colored solid

These extracts deliver extremely large amounts of THC to the body. Their use can send people to the emergency room for various reasons. The short-term effects of marijuana and concentrated TCH use include :

      altered senses (for example, seeing brighter colors)
      altered sense of time
      changes in mood
      impaired body movement
      difficulty with thinking and problem-solving
      impaired memory
      hallucinations (when taken in high doses)
      delusions (when taken in high doses)
      psychosis (risk is highest from high potency marijuana)

Another danger presented is when these extracts are prepared. The preparation of the materials usually involves butane, which is known generally as lighter fluid. Fires and explosions occur when the materials are being processed into the concentrated forms of the drug. People have been severely burned while using butane to make extracts in their own home.

The long-term effects of marijuana use are especially pernicious. Marijuana affects brain development of the young. It impairs brain activity of adults.

When people use marijuana during their teenage years, the drug may impair thinking, memory, and learning functions. It has a tendency to affect how the brain builds connections between the areas necessary for these functions.

People are still investigating how long marijuana's effects last and whether some changes may be permanent and irreversible. Following alcohol the most commonly used psychotropic drug in the United States is marijuana.

Its use is widespread among young Americans.

The rates of past year marijuana use among middle and high school students have remained at relatively the same level. A growing problem is that students in 8th and 10th grades who say they use it daily has grown considerably.
Vaping devices allow teenagers to start vaping concentrated THC. According to some survey each year 4% of 12th graders saying they vape THC daily.

An especially troubling belief is growing among the children themselves is that the use of these drugs is not harmful. In this case not only is the drug society raising and repeating these falsehoods but the large commercial companies that have entered the marijuana market have created a barrage of advertising and materials to support them.

People consume marijuana and its derivatives in various ways. They may smoke marijuana in hand-rolled, or manufactured cigarettes (joints) or through pipes or water pipes (known as bongs).

They may smoke it in emptied cigars that have been partly or completely refilled with marijuana – these are referred to as 'blunts'. In an attempt to avoid inhaling the smoke some users purchase various types of vaporizers. The vaporizers pull the active ingredients from the marijuana and concentrate their vapor in a small cell. A person then inhales the drugged mist in a concentrated form. Some vaporizers use a liquid marijuana extract.

Marijuana is mixed in foods which include, but are not limited to brownies, cookies, cakes and candy. Marijuana is boiled to make tea. THC-rich resins are also smoked or eaten directly.

CHAPTER 6

ALCOHOL USE

Alcohol Use

Drinking large amounts of alcohol once or on regular occasions can destroy a person's health and impact their mind.

Alcohol has different effects on different parts of the body :

With the brain alcohol breaks up the brain's communication system. It can affect the way the brain looks and works. Destruction like this can change mood and behavior in the short-term and with unpredictable changes over the long-term. Alcohol makes it difficult to think clearly and to move about normally.

For the heart drinking alcohol over a long time or too much on a single occasion can damage it and cause problems like :

Cardiomyopathy – Stretching and drooping of heart muscle
Arrhythmias – Irregular heart beat
Stroke
High blood pressure

The liver is especially sensitive to alcohol and its damage. Alcohol use hurts the liver and can lead to a many difficulties and liver inflammations including:

Steatosis, or fatty liver
Alcoholic hepatitis
Fibrosis
Cirrhosis

The pancreas is damaged as well. Alcohol forces the produce toxic substances that can lead to pancreatitis which is severe inflammation and swelling of the blood vessels in the pancreas that prevents proper digesting.

Alcohol can even lead to cancer.

There is strong scientific evidence of a link between drinking alcohol and different kinds of cancer. In just one report the evidence shows that the more alcohol someone consumes drinks the greater the risk of developing an alcohol-associated cancer.

Patterns between alcohol consumption and cancer are indicated for the following cancers :

"Head and neck cancer: Alcohol consumption is a major risk factor for certain head and neck cancers, particularly cancers of the oral cavity (excluding the lips), pharynx (throat), and larynx (voice box). People who consume 50 or more grams of alcohol per day (approximately 3.5 or more drinks per day) have at least a two to three times greater risk of developing these cancers than nondrinkers. Moreover, the risks of these cancers are substantially higher among persons who consume this amount of alcohol and also use tobacco.

Esophageal cancer: Alcohol consumption is a major risk factor for a particular type of esophageal cancer called esophageal squamous cell carcinoma. In addition, people who inherit a deficiency in an enzyme that metabolizes alcohol have been found to have substantially increased risks of alcohol-related esophageal squamous cell carcinoma.

Liver cancer: Alcohol consumption is an independent risk factor for, and a primary cause of, liver cancer (hepatocellular carcinoma). (Chronic infection with hepatitis B virus and hepatitis C virus are the other major causes of liver cancer.)

Breast cancer: More than 100 epidemiologic studies have looked at the association between alcohol consumption and the risk of breast cancer in women. These studies have consistently found an increased risk of breast cancer associated with increasing alcohol intake. A meta-analysis of 53 of these studies (which included a total of 58,000 women with breast cancer) showed that women who drank more than 45 grams of alcohol per day (approximately three drinks) had 1.5 times the risk of developing breast cancer as nondrinkers (a modestly increased risk). The risk of breast cancer was higher across all levels of alcohol intake: for every 10 grams of alcohol consumed per day (slightly less than one drink), researchers observed a small (7 percent) increase in the risk of breast cancer.

Colorectal cancer: Alcohol consumption is associated with a modestly increased risk of cancers of the colon and rectum. A meta-analysis of 57 cohort and case-control studiesthat examined the association between alcohol consumption and colorectal cancer risk showed that people who regularly drank 50 or more grams of alcohol per day (approximately 3.5 drinks) had 1.5 times the risk of developing colorectal cancer as nondrinkers or occasional drinkers. For every 10 grams of alcohol consumed per day, there was a small (7 percent) increase in the risk of colorectal cancer."

From the National Institute of Health :

"Drinking alcohol can weaken the immune system. This puts the body at a higher risk of disease. Long-term drinkers of alcohol are more liable to contract pneumonia and tuberculosis than people who do not Just drinking a lot of alcohol once slows your body's ability to ward off infections. This effect can last up to 24 hours after taking in the alcohol."

ABOUT THE AUTHOR

Alfred Brock was born in Flushing, New York in 1963
He loves his family very much
AB